SAXENDA

Dr. Dennis Reed

Saxenda

What is Saxenda?

Saxenda (liraglutide) is utilized for weight reduction and to assist with keeping weight off whenever weight has been lost, it is utilized for corpulent grown-ups or overweight grown-ups who likewise have weight-related clinical issues. Saxenda can be utilized in youngsters matured 12 to 17 years who with corpulence and who have a bodyweight over 132 pounds (60 kg). Saxenda is utilized along with a sound eating routine and exercise.

How does Saxenda function?

Saxenda attempts to assist with weighting misfortune by bringing down hunger, easing back gastric exhausting which encourages you for longer and accordingly you decline your calorie admission. Saxenda is like a chemical that happens normally in the body and assists control with blooding sugar, insulin levels, and processing. Saxenda has a place with a class of meds called glucagon-like peptide-1 (GLP-1) agonists.

Saxenda incidental effects

Gets crisis clinical assistance assuming you have indications of a hypersensitive response to Saxenda: hives; quick pulses; dizziness; inconvenience breathing or gulping; face lips, tongue, or throat swelling

Gallbladder issues - fever, upper stomach torment, earth shaded stools, jaundice (yellowing of your skin or eyes);

Side effects of pancreatitis - serious agony in your upper stomach spreading to your back, queasiness regardless of spewing, quick pulse;

seriously low glucose - outrageous shortcoming, disarray, quakes, perspiring, quick pulse, inconvenience talking, queasiness, heaving, fast breathing, swooning, and seizure (spasms); or on the other hand

Kidney issues - practically no pee; excruciating or troublesome pee; expanding in your feet or lower legs; feeling drained or winded.

Three Canadian patient associations — Weight Canada, Diabetes Canada, and the Gastrointestinal (GI) Society — gave contribution to this accommodation. Weight Canada will be Canada's driving stoutness enrolled foundation relationship for experts and patients, contributing exploration, schooling, and backing for Canadians living with heftiness.

Diabetes Canada is a national health charity that focuses on population-level research and policy initiatives for diabetes prevention, care, and cure. It represents Canadians with diabetes or at risk for developing it. The GI Society is a public cause focused on working on the existences of individuals with GI and liver circumstances through research, pushing for expanded admittance to medical services, and advancing GI and liver wellbeing.

Heftiness Canada directed patient meetings and an internet based overview, where 5 of the people talked with and 60% of the review respondents had utilized liraglutide 3 mg for stoutness the executives. Diabetes Canada submitted patient information utilizing information from 2 web-based overviews led in July and August 2020 and in December 2020 and January 2021.

The GI Society utilized information from patient and patient guardian meets, the consequences of distributed investigations, and a study directed from October 6, 2020, to January 10, 2021, among people living with corpulence. Every one of the 3 patient information bunches submitted irreconcilable circumstance divulgences, which can be found on the CADTH site.

According to patient groups, obesity is associated with inequality in access to employment, health care, and education as well as an increase in the likelihood of developing additional diseases.

The GI Society revealed that 72% of their study respondent's experienced social disgrace because of living with stoutness, with many detailing that they try not to get clinical consideration since they feel like their doctor disgraces them due to their weight. People living with weight likewise report dissatisfaction with the effect that the constant and frequently misjudged infection has on their general personal satisfaction.

At present, most Canadians living with corpulence revealed utilizing diet and exercise, drugs, or bariatric medical procedure to battle the sickness. A lot of people who exercise and diet have trouble keeping up their efforts or finding a program that works for them, which can cause depression, hopelessness, and more weight gain. Supported prescriptions incorporate NB (Contrave), liraglutide (Saxenda), and orlistat (Xenical), all of which make unfortunate side impacts. Notwithstanding the accessibility of these medications, the GI Society detailed many worries about getting and paying for the remedies of these medications.

Patient gatherings revealed that numerous patients would like a treatment that is powerful in the long haul, is reasonable, and makes no or negligible side impacts. Patient gatherings trust that liraglutide 3 mg might assist individuals with bettering deal with their weight, possibly postponing or forestalling the improvement of comorbidities, for example, the movement of prediabetes to type 2 diabetes.

Besides, when gotten some information about results to consider, it was accounted for that patients zeroed in less on better weight than on superior wellbeing related comorbidities (e.g., diabetes, hypertension, and rest apnea) as well as results connected with regular day to day existence, for example, efficiency, energy levels, rest, action, and psychological well-being.

Clinician Info

The clinical master counseled for this survey noticed that aftereffects limit the utilization of each of the 3 pharmacotherapies endorsed in Canada, for certain patients expecting to stop the prescription totally because of secondary effects. The medical professional acknowledged that medications for obesity typically result in weight loss of 5 to 10 percent, which is considered sufficient to alleviate weight-related comorbidities like type 2 diabetes and osteoarthritis. In any case, in an ideal world, we would have pharmacotherapy that advances bigger measures of weight reduction.

The master showed that as per the Heftiness Canada 2020 rules, pharmacotherapy can practically be utilized anyplace in a patient's weight the board venture. Further, albeit the master showed that it is sensible for a patient to attempt way of life mediation first prior to beginning liraglutide 3 mg, that approach isn't required, especially for patients at higher BMIs. Since the component of activity is altogether different from NB and orlistat, a few doctors are endorsing blends of these specialists for weight reduction, regardless of insignificant proof to help this.

The clinical master expressed that at present, it is basically impossible to anticipate which patients will lose the most weight with liraglutide, yet that passing patients can be recognized utilizing the customary meaning of overweight and heftiness in view of BMI classification. Patients with Class III obesity (i.e., BMI > 40 kg/m2), those with Edmonton Obesity Staging System (EOSS) scores ranging from EOSS 1 to EOSS 3, and those with the highest prevalence of weight-related comorbidities are the most in need of weight loss intervention.

The clinical master counseled for this survey expressed that as a general rule, weight reduction results are evaluated in view of progress in BMI and weight, while weight-related comorbidity results are assessed involving change in boundaries, for example, circulatory strain, glycemic control, and lipid profile. After 12 to 16 weeks at the maximum dose, along with behavioral and lifestyle changes, weight loss response is evaluated to determine whether the medication should be continued at that point. The master showed that most doctors would concur that a 5% to 10% complete body weight reduction is clinically significant and is ordinarily felt to be related with worked on metabolic boundaries. The expert stated, based on previous experience, that once the patient is successful on a stable dose of liraglutide 3 mg, assessments may be spaced out over three months, eventually becoming every six months.

Drug Program Info

The medication plans mentioned explanation in regards to the potential objective patient populace and the expected treatment length of liraglutide. The clinical master thought about that it would be sensible to consider pharmacotherapy in patients with a BMI between 27 kg/m2 and 30 kg/m2 without comorbidity as second-line after way of life changes, albeit this would be past the Wellbeing Canada-endorsed sign. The master felt that patients would recapture the weight they had lost assuming pharmacologic treatment for weight the board was stopped; accordingly, such medicines would should be gone on in the long haul, even in patients whose BMI dipped under 30 kg/m2 (or 27 kg/m2 in patients with weight-related comorbidities). The public medication designs additionally mentioned explanation in regards to re-treatment in patients who recapture weight, or on the other hand if liraglutide 3 mg becomes inadequate over the long haul after an underlying wanted reaction. According to the clinical expert, a patient is unlikely to respond better to weight loss medication in the future if there is no benefit after the first attempt. As a result, it is highly unlikely that the drug will be prescribed to that patient again for the same purpose.

Albeit every one of the preliminaries were twofold visually impaired randomized examinations with a fake treatment control bunch, the extent of patients who suspended rashly was high in the investigations in general, bringing about critical measures of missing information, which were credited utilizing last perception conveyed forward (LOCF). Nonetheless, the higher pace of end because of AEs and the tremendous contrast in weight reduction with liraglutide 3 mg contrasted and fake treatment, as well as the bigger extent of patients who ceased the concentrate because of inadequate treatment in the fake treatment bunch, may have brought about unblinding for certain patients.

In every one of the preliminaries, factual testing strategies depended on the essential end point with the end goal that the assurance of review power and test sizes didn't think about optional results. Hence, there is a gamble of type I mistake expansion in key results like HRQoL, glycemic control, and weight-related CV comorbidities. In addition, the study permitted the recalculation of dietary portions based on a patient's response to treatment after 28 weeks. In any case, there was no information to freely confirm how frequently the eating regimen changes occurred and in the event that they happened in a fair way across treatment gatherings. It means a lot to take note of that considering the basic significance of calorie admission to weight the board, unevenness in this part of the co-mediation can possibly shift the results for 1 gathering over the other.

In every one of the preliminaries, patients inside the BMI section of 30 kg/m2 to 40 kg/m2 or more represented over 85% of the review populace. This shows that a gathering of patients determined in the sign (i.e., patients who are overweight with a BMI of 27 kg/m2 to less than 30 kg/m2 with comorbidities) was not enough addressed in any of the examinations.

Further, the preliminaries enlisted prevalently White patients (72% to 88%) and in 3 of the examinations, the patients were generally ladies (54% to 78%). As per the clinical master counseled in this audit, the review populace doesn't mirror the identity blend of patients who are overweight or living with stoutness in Canada. Likewise, the high extent of ladies in the review populaces varies from the 67% pace of heftiness in grown-up guys in Canada, as revealed by CTFPHC.4 The prohibition models denied passage to certain patients, for example, those taking drugs that causes weight gain and those recovering load after a past bariatric medical procedure, who might be viewed as clinically pertinent patients and who might require pharmacotherapy for constant weight the board. It is unknown how much these issues affect the generalizability of the findings that were reported.

Relevant to this review were two additional comparative RCTs comparing liraglutide 3 mg with intensive lifestyle intervention. The two preliminaries give extra proof of liraglutide 3 mg contrasted and escalated way of life change, which was recognized as a comparator of interest in the CADTH survey convention.

Study 4274 was a planned, multi-focus, twofold visually impaired, fake treatment controlled, stage IIIb randomized preliminary to assess the medical advantages of consolidating serious social treatment (IBT) with liraglutide 3 mg in grown-up patients living with corpulence without diabetes, and Study NCT02911818 was a solitary site, open-mark, equal gathering randomized preliminary to survey whether the expansion of liraglutide 3 mg to an IBT mediation would increment weight reduction contrasted with IBT alone in grown-up patients living with heftiness.

Across the 2 investigations, a sum of 432 patients was haphazardly doled out to be treated with liraglutide 3 mg or fake treatment. The members were dominatingly female (79% to 84%) and the mean period of patients was between 45 years and 49 years. The patients in Study 4274 were for the most part White (79% and 82% for the liraglutide 3 mg and fake treatment gatherings, separately), though for Study NCT02911818, 54.0% self-distinguished as non-Hispanic White, 44.7% as Dark, and 6.7% as Hispanic. Generally speaking, benchmark attributes seemed comparable for the treatment gatherings of each review. In any case, in Study 4274, the liraglutide 3 mg bunch had a more noteworthy extent of patients with a BMI of 40 kg/m2 or more than the fake treatment bunch (40.8% versus 30.7%).

In the two preliminaries, liraglutide 3 mg was utilized as an assistant to the US Places for Federal medical insurance and Medicaid Administrations (CMS)- IBT (CMS-IBT) at the endorsed portion and following suggested titration methodologies recently depicted. The CMS-IBT comprised of week after week, 15-minute, in-person way of life directing visits the main month, trailed by visits each and every other week the following 5 months, approximating 14 contacts to 15 contacts north of a half year along with expanded actual work and explicit day to day energy consumption in view of patients' weight. In Study 4274, the comparator was fake treatment in addition to CMS-IBT, while in Study NCT02911818; the comparator was CMS-IBT alone.

Concentrate on 4274 had 2 co-essential end focuses: the percentage of patients who have lost at least 5% of their baseline weight by week 56, as well as the change in body weight (%) from baseline to week 56. The essential end point of Study NCT02911818 was the mean rate decrease in standard body weight at week 52.

Liraglutide, the second GLP-1 simple endorsed in 2009 in Europe and 2010 in USA under the business trademark Victoza (Novo Nordisk). Liraglutide is a manufactured particle delivered utilizing DNA recombinant innovation. Contrasted with local GLP-1, it has an expansion of a 16 carbon unsaturated fat side-chain at Lys26 and an Arg34Lys replacement (Neumiller et al., 2010). After s.d. infusion, just 1-2% of liraglutide flows as free peptide in the plasma as the rest is no covalently bound to egg whites as guaranteed by the unsaturated fat side-chain (Zhang et al., 2012).

Liraglutide's half-life is increased to 11–15 hours as a result, necessitating daily administration. A beginning portion of 0.6 mg/portion is suggested for multi week, and on the off chance that very much endured, it is expanded to 1.2 mg/portion. The measurements can additionally be expanded to 1.8 mg/portion whenever required. A clinical preliminary program called Liraglutide Impact and Activity in Diabetes (LEAD) concentrated on the viability of liraglutide (Buse et al., 2009, 2010b; 2009 et al., 2009; Nauck et al., 2009; Russell-Jones et al., 2009; Zinman et al., 2009). HbA1c, FPG, and body weight levels were fundamentally diminished by 0.8-1.5%,

2.6 mM, and 2-3 kg, separately, in Liraglutide bunches when contrasted with fake treatment. 1.7-2.5 mM decrease in PPG trips in liraglutide treatment bunches is credited with its impact on gastric discharging (Degn et al., 2004). In addition, event of hypoglycemia was low. A 26-week randomized, global, open-mark, equal gathering study was directed by Buse and collaborators, which looked at the impact of liraglutide on a no holds barred preliminary with that of exenatide and Lixisenatide (Buse et al., 2009; Kapitza and other, 2013). Liraglutide achieved more decreases in HbA1c levels contrasted with that of exenatide (1.1% versus 0.8%)

alongside better control in FPG (1.6 versus 0.6 mM) (Buse et al., 2009). Exenatide then again would do well to control in PPG after breakfast and supper contrasted with liraglutide (1.9 versus 1.3 mM). Both exenatide and liraglutide performed similarly in body weight decrease. When contrasted and lixisenatide, liraglutide performed better in diminishing HbA1c level (0.3% versus 0.5%) and FPG level (0.3 versus 1.3 mM) while lixisenatide performed better in lessening PPG journey after breakfast. Liraglutide achieved critical decreases in body weight decrease (2.4 versus 1.6 kg) too when contrasted with lixisenatide (Kapitza et al., 2013).

Restricting to egg whites impedes renal disposal, giving liraglutide a half-existence of roughly 12 h. The sluggish retention of liraglutide from subcutaneous tissues delivers a most extreme blood fixation after 8-12 h, subsequently allowing once-everyday infusion. It is hypothesized that staying away from pinnacles of the medication assists with lessening the trademark gastrointestinal aftereffects.

In the UK, liraglutide is supported for the treatment of grown-ups with type 2 diabetes in mix with metformin or a sulfonylurea, in mix with metformin and a sulfonylurea, or added to metformin and a thiazolidinedione.

Liraglutide is formed as an answer for subcutaneous infusion in pre-filled pens conveying 0.6, 1.2 or 1.8 mg per portion. The proposed beginning portion is 0.6 mg day to day, expanding after at least seven days to the support portion of 1.2 mg day to day. After essentially one more week, the portion can be expanded to 1.8 mg whenever required, albeit this portion isn't suggested by the UK's Public Establishment of Wellbeing and Clinical Greatness (NICE).

The organization has likewise indicated standards that ought to provoke surrender of treatment in view of a blend of weight decrease and glycemic impacts; these limitations additionally apply to exenatide in the UK. Alternate glucose-lowering medications should be taken into consideration if an inadequate response is observed after six months of treatment. Utilization of liraglutide isn't suggested in patients with moderate levels of renal disability, for example where creatinine freedom is 30-60 ml/min. Liraglutide has not been concentrated on in patients with seriously weakened renal capability, and information in patients with hepatic hindrance are restricted.

In patients with type 2 diabetes liraglutide can fundamentally bring down HbA1c with associative enhancements in fasting and postprandial blood glucose levels. Dose-dependent weight loss ranges from about 1 to 3 kg. The really unfriendly occasions are sickness and loose bowels, albeit the recurrence of gastrointestinal aftereffects will frequently diminish over the long haul. Bringing down of fatty substances and decreases in pulse have likewise been noticed.

Diet and Weight reduction

It's a well-known fact that America has a weight issue. Nearly three-quarters of us are overweight or obese, according to the CDC. However in excess of 160 million Americans are on a tight eating routine at some random time, and we drop more than $70 billion every year on business weight reduction plans, supplements and other pound-shedding measures. That recommends that terrible weight is difficult — yet it is not outside the realm of possibilities when done well. There are two keys to progress with regards to weight reduction. The first is to find a methodology that works for you explicitly, one that causes you to feel quite a bit better and keeps you inspired. The second is to take as much time as necessary — manageable weight reduction happens gradually however consistently.

What's the best eating regimen for weight reduction?

After deciding that they need to lose some weight, the most common question is, "What is the best diet for weight loss?" That's not a stupid question, but it often suggests a less-than-ideal strategy, such as planning to eat extremely restrictively for a while until the weight is lost before returning to normal eating. People who have lost weight and maintained it typically have made a permanent shift toward healthier eating habits rather than adhering to "fad diets." You will be able to lose weight and enjoy numerous other advantages by simply substituting healthy foods for unhealthy ones—not just for a few weeks but for the rest of your life. So a superior arrangement of inquiries may be, "What is a sound eating routine? What does a solid eating routine resemble?"

A sound eating regimen favors regular, natural food varieties over pre-bundled feasts and tidbits. It is adjusted, implying that it furnishes your body with every one of the supplements and minerals it necessities to work best. It stresses plant-based food sources — particularly products of the soil — over creature food sources. It contains a lot of protein. It is low in sugar and salt. It integrates "solid fats" including fish, olive oil and other plant-determined oils.

Here are a few examples of weight loss-friendly meals. For breakfast, a bowl of wheat chips with cut strawberries and pecans with nonfat milk. For lunch, a turkey sandwich on wheat with vegetables and an olive oil and vinegar dressing. A salmon steak served with spinach for dinner.

What's the best eating regimen?

There is no single eating regimen that nutritionists have considered "the best." Nonetheless, there are a few styles of eating that specialists either have intended for ideal wellbeing or have seen to be solid when consumed customarily by various individuals all over the planet. Such styles of eating will generally share a couple of things for all intents and purpose — they will generally be plant-based counts calories, they underscore solid fats, no straightforward sugars and low sodium, and they favor regular food sources over the exceptionally handled charge run of the mill of a large part of the Western eating routine.

For instance, the Mediterranean style diet gets its name from the food sources accessible to different societies situated around the Mediterranean Ocean. It emphasizes whole grains, legumes, fruits, and vegetables that have been minimally processed. It has fish, yogurt, cheese, and poultry in moderate amounts. Olive oil is its essential cooking fat. Red meat and food varieties with added sugars are just eaten sparingly. Other than being a successful weight reduction technique, eating a Mediterranean style diet is connected to a lower hazard of coronary illness, diabetes, discouragement and a few types of malignant growth.

Specialists fostered the Scramble diet (Dietary Ways to deal with Stop Hypertension) explicitly as a heart-solid routine. The blend of food types contained in the eating regimen appear to cooperate particularly really to bring down pulse and lessening hazard of cardiovascular breakdown. DASH is characterized by a low level of saturated fat and cholesterol, a high intake of potassium, magnesium, calcium, fiber, and magnesium, and little to no red meat or sugar. That amounts to a list of foods that are similar to the Mediterranean diet—whole grains, vegetables, fruits, fish, poultry, nuts, and olive oil—which is not surprising.

The Mediterranean-DASH diet Intervention for Neurodegenerative Delay, also known as the MIND diet, was developed by medical professionals to incorporate aspects of the Mediterranean and DASH diets that appeared to improve brain health and prevent cognitive decline and dementia.

Practically speaking, it is basically the same as both the Mediterranean and Run counts calories, yet it puts more grounded accentuation on verdant green vegetables and berries, and less accentuation on leafy foods.

Lately, the Nordic eating regimen has arisen as both a weight reduction and wellbeing support diet. In view of Scandinavian eating designs, the Nordic eating regimen is weighty on fish, apples, and pears, entire grains like rye and oats, and cold-environment vegetables including cabbage, carrots and cauliflower. Studies have upheld its utilization both in forestalling stroke and in weight reduction.

What do these eating regimens share practically speaking? They're great overall for your heart, they all comprise of normal natural food varieties and they all contain a lot of plant-based dishes. Eating for your wellbeing — particularly your heart wellbeing — by taking on components from these eating regimens is a shrewd method for getting thinner.

What is irregular fasting?

Intermittent fasting success stories are probably something you've heard of. Be that as it may, is fasting solid, and does discontinuous fasting work?

Fasting, or abstaining from food for a certain amount of time, is an ancient practice that is safe if not used to its full potential. Customarily, the advantages of fasting have been both otherworldly and physical. Individuals who quick for strict reasons frequently report a more grounded center around otherworldly issues during the quick. Genuinely, a basic quick brings down glucose, diminishes irritation, further develops digestion, cleans out poisons off of harmed cells and has been connected to bring down chance of malignant growth, decreased torment from joint pain and upgraded cerebrum capability.

Discontinuous fasting implies splitting one's time between "eating windows" and times of abstention consistently. A typical intermittent fasting schedule might limit eating to 7:00 a.m. to 3:00 p.m., and the remaining 16 hours of the day might be spent fasting. In any case, there is no particular, endorsed plan. Some people have eating windows that are either more or less generous. For example, they say they won't eat after 8:00 p.m., or they only let themselves eat every other day.

The science behind irregular fasting depends on modifying the body's digestion. During a period without eating, insulin levels drop to the point that the body starts consuming fat for fuel. Furthermore, the reasoning goes, by easing back the body's digestion; you make your hunger drop off and hence will consume less calories when you continue eating.

Various examinations have shown the advantages of irregular fasting for weight reduction. Nonetheless, obviously it is any more compelling than essentially confining calories and following a typical eating plan. One potential justification for the outcome of discontinuous fasting is that most specialists have stopped the propensity for eating during the late night and night hours. Limiting eating to prior in the day adjusts better to our bodies' circadian rhythms and is less inclined to make us store our food in fat cells. Since discontinuous fasting is challenging for some individuals to stick to, a savvy option may be to consume a low-calorie Mediterranean eating routine and to stop the day's eating in late evening.

If you have diabetes or heart disease, for example, you shouldn't try intermittent fasting without first talking to your doctor.

Discontinuous fasting is a very "way of life escalated" dietary example, implying that keeping up with despite ordinary social relationships is testing. Assuming that the remainder of your family is eating while you're fasting, you may be enticed to enjoy or to give up the family-feast custom. On the off chance that your occupation expects you to eat with clients or associates, you'll find an irregular fasting plan hard to keep up with. Recollect that the best good dieting plan is the one you'll adhere to.

What's a high-fat weight reduction diet?

It sounds strange, yet many individuals make progress getting in shape — particularly at first — by eating more fat, not less. Called a ketogenic or Keto diet, this strategy requires moving the primary wellspring of calories over to greasy food sources — somewhere in the range of 75% and 90% of what you eat, with just 10-20% of your calories coming from protein and a simple 5% from starches. The hypothesis is that by eating such countless sound fats and confining carbs, you enter an adjusted metabolic state where you force your body to start depending on fat for energy, consuming with extreme heat your fat stores rather than sugar for fuel.

Research shows that keto is a compelling method for hopping start weight reduction and further develop glucose levels. In any case, it is difficult to keep up with, and to date we are missing long haul concentrates on that demonstrate it to be a reasonable eating design for keeping weight off.

What does a Good dieting Plate resemble?

Since both weight reduction and by and large wellbeing are attached to some fundamental eating designs, we have fostered the Harvard Good dieting Plate as a model for dinner arranging and for your generally speaking adjusted diet. Envision a round supper plate with a line running upward down its middle partitioning it uniformly in two. One portion of the plate ought to be taken up by equivalent parts of entire grains (not refined grains like white bread and white rice) and sound protein (like fish, nuts, beans and poultry — not red meat or handled meats). Fruit should make up the remaining portion, while vegetables should make up two-thirds of the remaining portion. Attempt to infuse a great deal of assortment into this portion of your plate (or a big part of your eating routine) — eat natural products in various varieties and vegetables of different types (yet don't count potatoes or French fries as vegetables).

For beforehand stationary people, a sluggish movement in actual work has been suggested so 30 minutes of work-out every day is accomplished following half a month of steady development. This may likewise apply to some tactical work force, particularly newcomers or reservists reviewed to deployment ready who might be entering administration from already exceptionally inactive ways of life.

The action objective has been communicated as an expansion in energy use of 1,000 kcal/wk (Jakicic et al., 1999; Pate et al., 1995), even though this amount might not be enough to stop weight gain. For that reason, a week by week objective of 2,000 to 3,000 kcal of added action might be essential (Klem et al., 1997; Schoeller et al., 1997). In this manner, mental groundwork for how much action important to keep up with weight reduction should start while getting thinner (Brownell, 1999).

For some people, changing action levels is seen as more horrendous than addressing dietary propensities. It has been demonstrated that dividing a 30-minute daily exercise "prescription" into 10-minute bouts increases compliance more than longer bouts (Jakicic et al., 1995, Pate et al., 1995).

Nonetheless, north of an 18-month time span, people who performed short episodes of actual work didn't encounter enhancements in long haul weight reduction, cardiorespiratory wellness, or actual work cooperation in correlation with the people who performed longer episodes of activity. Some proof proposes that home gym equipment (e.g., a treadmill) improves the probability of standard activity and is related with more noteworthy long haul weight reduction (Jakicic et al., 1999). What's more, individual inclinations are fundamental contemplations in decisions of action.

While strength preparing or opposition practice is joined with vigorous movement, long haul results might be preferable over those with heart stimulating exercise alone (Poirier and Despres, 2001; Sothern et al., 1999). The loss of lean body mass may be minimized and the relative loss of body fat may be increased as a result of strength training's tendency to build muscle. An additional advantage is the weakening of the diminishing in resting metabolic rate related with weight reduction, conceivably as a result of protecting or upgrading lean weight.

However important as exercise seems to be, the current examination writing on overweight people shows that exercise programs alone don't deliver critical weight reduction in the populaces considered. It ought to be stressed, in any case, that an enormous number of such examinations have been led with moderately aged Caucasian ladies driving stationary ways of life. The disappointment of activity alone to create critical weight reduction might be on the grounds that the neurochemical systems that control eating conduct make people make up for the calories consumed in practice by expanding food (calorie) admission. While practice projects can bring about a normal weight reduction of 2 to 3 kg temporarily (Blair, 1993; Pavlou et al., 1989a; Skender et al., 1996; Wadden and Sarwer, 1999), result improves altogether when active work is joined with dietary mediation. For instance, when actual work was joined with a decreased calorie diet and way of life change, a weight reduction of 7.2 kg was accomplished following a half year to 3 years of follow-up (Blair, 1993).

Actual work in addition to abstain from food delivers improved results than one or the other eating routine or active work alone (Blair, 1993; Dyer, 1994; Pavlou et al., 1989a, 1989b; Perri et al., 1993). Furthermore, weight recapture is fundamentally more outlandish when actual work is joined with some other weight-decrease routine (Blair, 1993; Klem et al., 1997). Proceeded trail closely behind weight reduction is related with further developed result in the event that the movement plan is checked and changed as a component of this development (Kayman et al., 1990).

The fact that people become or remain overweight as a result of modifiable habits or behaviors (see Chapter 3) and that weight loss and weight maintenance can be achieved by changing those behaviors is the foundation for the use of behavior and lifestyle modification in weight management. The essential objectives of conduct procedures for weight control are to increment active work and to diminish caloric admission by adjusting dietary patterns (Brownell and Kramer, 1994; Wilson, 1995).

A subcategory of change in conduct, ecological administration, is examined in the following segment. Social treatment, which was presented during the 1960s, might be given to a solitary individual or to gatherings of clients. Commonly, people partake in 12 to 20 week after week meetings that last from 1 to 2 hours each (Brownell and Kramer, 1994), with an objective of weight reduction in the scope of 1 to 2 lb/wk (Brownell and Kramer, 1994). Previously, social methodologies were applied as independent medicines to just change dietary patterns and decrease caloric admission. Notwithstanding, more as of late, these therapies have been utilized in blend with low-calorie eats less, clinical nourishment treatment, sustenance schooling, practice programs, checking, pharmacological specialists, and social help to advance weight reduction, and as a part of upkeep programs.

A few extra methods remembered for social therapy programs incorporate eating just routinely planned feasts; doing nothing else while eating; consuming dinners just in one spot (typically the lounge area) and leaving the table in the wake of eating; shopping just from a rundown; and going shopping after having eaten a lot (Brownell and Kramer, 1994).

A crucial component of the behavioral treatment of overweight and obesity is also the use of reinforcement strategies. According to Brownell and

Kramer (1994), subjects may choose a positive event, such as participating in a particularly enjoyable activity or purchasing a special item when a goal is achieved.

Cognitive restructuring of erroneous or dysfunctional beliefs regarding weight regulation may be another important component of behavioral treatment programs (Wing, 1998). Methods created by mental conduct specialists can be utilized to assist the person with distinguishing explicit triggers for gorging, manage pessimistic perspectives towards stoutness in the public eye, and understand that a minor dietary infraction doesn't mean disappointment. Nourishment training and social help, talked about later in this part, are additionally parts of conduct programs.

Conduct medicines of weight are much of the time effective temporarily. In any case, the drawn out adequacy of these medicines is more disputable, with information recommending that numerous people return to their underlying body weight inside 3 to 5

Ongoing investigations of people who have made progress at long haul weight reduction might offer different experiences into ways of further developing social treatment procedures. Klem and colleagues (1997) discovered in their analysis of data from the National Weight Control Registry that weight loss that is achieved through exercise, sensible dieting, consuming less fat, and individual behavior changes can be maintained for long periods of time. In any case, this populace was self-chosen so it doesn't address the experience of the typical individual in a non-military personnel populace.

Since they have accomplished and kept a lot of weight reduction (no less than 30 lb for at least 2 years), there is motivation to accept that the populace signed up for the Vault might be particularly focused. In that capacity, the experience of individuals in the Library might give knowledge into the tactical populace, despite the fact that proof to declare this with power is deficient. Anyway, most of members in the Library report they have rolled out critical extremely durable improvements in their way of behaving, including segment control, low-fat food choice, at least 60 minutes of everyday work-out, self-checking, and very much leveled up critical thinking abilities.

The time it takes to complete a task and the inaccessibility of facilities or safe places to exercise are major obstacles to exercise, even for highly motivated individuals. Natural mediations underscore the numerous ways that actual work can be squeezed into a bustling way of life and look to create utilization of anything that open doors are accessible (HHS, 1996). Ecological changes might be expected to empower female cooperation in practice programs, like convenience of the requirement for more after-work out "fix time" by ladies and worksite offices that are more "easy to understand, for example, estimated indoor strolling courses and noon low-level vigorous exercise classes (Wasserman et al., 2000). The accessibility of safe walkways and parks and elective techniques for transportation to work, like strolling or bicycling, additionally upgrade the active work climate. Laying out "vehicle free" zones is an illustration of an ecological change that could advance expanded actual work.

Nourishment Instruction

The board of overweight and corpulence requires the dynamic investment of the person. Nourishment experts can give people a base of data that permits them to go with educated food decisions.

Nourishment schooling is unmistakable from sustenance directing, albeit the items cross-over impressively. Sustenance guiding and dietary administration will generally zero in more straightforwardly on the persuasive, close to home, and mental issues related with the ongoing errand of weight reduction and weight the executives. It tends to the how of conduct changes in the dietary field. Sustenance schooling then again, gives essential data about the logical groundwork of nourishment that empowers individuals to settle on informed conclusions about food, cooking strategies, eating out, and assessing segment sizes. Sustenance training programs likewise may give data on the job of nourishment in wellbeing advancement and sickness counteraction, sports sustenance, and nourishment for pregnant and lactating ladies. Knowledge of nutrition and its application to healthy living is passed on through effective nutrition education. For instance, it makes sense of the idea of energy balance in weight the board in an available, useful way that has significance to the singular's way of life, remembering that for the tactical setting.

Composed materials arranged by different government offices or by charitable wellbeing associations can be utilized actually to give nourishment instruction. In any case, composed materials are best when used to support casual homeroom or guiding meetings and to give explicit data, for example, a table of the calorie content of food varieties. The arrangement of schooling programs shifts significantly, and can incorporate conventional classes, casual gathering gatherings, or remotely coordinating. A typical foundation among bunch individuals is useful (however rare conceivable).

Instructive organizations that give down to earth and important sustenance data for program members are the best. For instance, some tactical weight-the executives programs incorporate field outings to post trades, cafés (inexpensive food and others), motion pictures, and different spots where food is bought or eaten (Vorachek, 1999).

The association of life partners and other relatives in a schooling program improves the probability that different individuals from the family will roll out long-lasting improvements, which thus upgrades the probability that the program members will keep on getting in shape or keep up with weight reduction (Hart et al., 1990; Hertzler and Schulman, 1983; Sperry, 1985).

Specific consideration should be coordinated to contribution of those in the family who are probably going to look for and get ready food. Except if the program member lives alone, sustenance the board is seldom viable without the contribution of relatives.

Healthfully Adjusted, Hypocaloric Diets

A healthfully adjusted, hypocaloric diet has been the proposal of most dietitians who are directing patients who wish to get in shape. This sort of diet is made out of the kinds of food varieties a patient generally eats, however in lower amounts. There are various reasons such eating regimens are engaging, however the fundamental explanation is that the proposal is straightforward — people need just to follow the U.S. Branch of Horticulture's Food Guide Pyramid.

www.ingramcontent.com/pod-product-compliance
Lightning Source LLC
Chambersburg PA
CBHW071016290526
45795CB00005B/1821